GESTATIONAL DIABETES RECIPES FOR VEGETARIANS

Nourishing Vegetarian Meals for a Healthy Gestational Journey

T. John

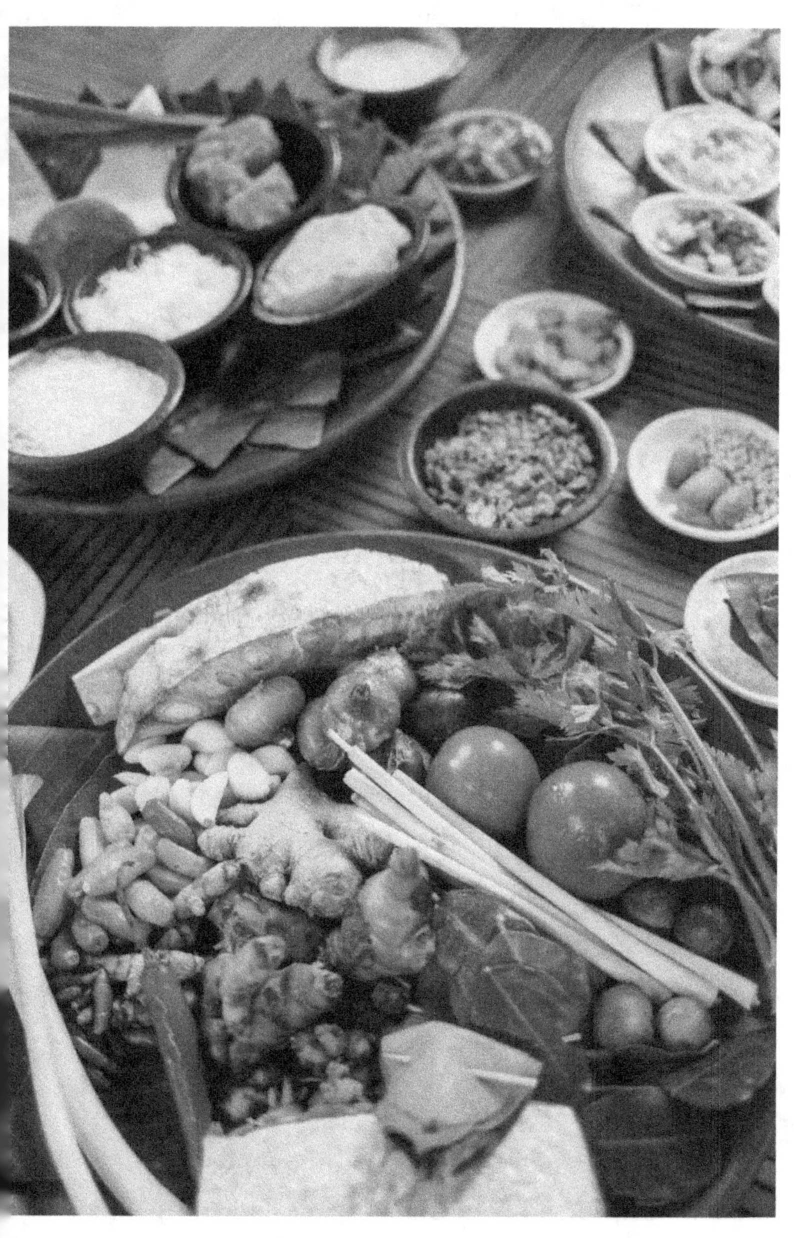

TABLE OF CONTENTS

Chapter 3: Lunch Recipes..46

Chapter 6: Desserts 114

Chapter 7: Smoothies 137

CONCLUSION .... 15?

INTRODUCTION

Congratulations on your pregnancy! It's an exciting time, filled with anticipation and maybe a few jitters. One condition that can arise during pregnancy is gestational diabetes (GDM). While it sounds scary, informed choices and a focus on healthy eating can help you manage it effectively. Let's delve into understanding GDM, the importance of diet management, and how vegetarianism can play a role in this journey.

Understanding Gestational Diabetes:

Imagine your body is a grand bakery, churning out energy for you and your growing baby. Insulin, a hormone, acts like the key, unlocking your cells to absorb this energy (sugar) from the bloodstream. During pregnancy, your placenta can sometimes produce substances that interfere with insulin, leading to high blood sugar levels – that's gestational diabetes.

Why is Diet Management Important?

Uncontrolled GDM can pose risks for both you and your baby. It can increase the chance of excessive weight gain in your baby, leading to delivery complications. Fortunately, managing your blood sugar levels through diet is a powerful tool.

The Power of Plate Planning:

Think of your plate as a colorful canvas. Here's a breakdown of what to include:

- **Colorful Veggies:** They're packed with fiber, which helps regulate blood sugar absorption. Think leafy greens, broccoli, and peppers.
- **Lean Protein:** It keeps you feeling full and provides essential nutrients for you and your baby. Choose options like fish, beans, tofu, or lentils.
- **Healthy Fats:** Don't ditch all fats! Avocados, nuts, and seeds offer healthy fats that keep you satiated and support fetal development.

- **Whole Grains:** Brown rice, quinoa, and whole-wheat bread provide sustained energy without spiking your blood sugar.

Can a Vegetarian Diet Help?

Vegetarian diets, rich in fiber and naturally lower in saturated fat, can be a great foundation for managing GDM. However, a few things to consider:

- **Planning is Key:** A well-planned vegetarian diet can ensure you get all the essential nutrients, including iron and vitamin B12, which are crucial during pregnancy. Consult a registered dietitian to craft a personalized plan.

- **Focus on Variety:** Explore the diverse world of vegetarian protein sources – lentils, chickpeas, tofu, tempeh, and a variety of nuts and seeds.

- **Don't Forget Dairy (or Alternatives):** Calcium is vital for your baby's bone development. Include low-fat dairy products or calcium-fortified plant-based alternatives in your diet.

Remember:

- You're Not Alone: Many women manage GDM with a healthy diet and support from their healthcare team.
- Small Changes, Big Impact: Start with incorporating small changes and gradually build a sustainable eating pattern.
- Celebrate Milestones: Be proud of your healthy choices and the positive impact they have on you and your baby.

By understanding GDM and embracing a dietary approach that works for you, vegetarian or not, you can navigate your pregnancy with confidence and ensure a healthy journey for both you and your little one.

Chapter 1: 30 Day Meal Plan

Week 1:

Day 1:

- Breakfast: Quinoa Breakfast Bowl
- Lunch: Lentil and Vegetable Soup
- Dinner: Cauliflower Rice Stir Fry
- Snack: Guacamole with Veggie Sticks
- Dessert: Berry Crisp with Oat Topping

Day 2:

- Breakfast: Avocado Toast with Chickpeas
- Lunch: Caprese Salad with Balsamic Glaze
- Dinner: Eggplant Parmesan
- Snack: Hummus and Whole Grain Crackers
- Dessert: Chocolate Avocado Mousse

Day 3:

- Breakfast: Vegetable Omelette
- Lunch: Chickpea Salad with Lemon Tahini Dressing
- Dinner: Butternut Squash Risotto

- Snack: Roasted Chickpeas
- Dessert: Banana Bread with Walnuts

Day 4:

- Breakfast: Chia Seed Pudding with Berries
- Lunch: Grilled Vegetable Wrap with Hummus
- Dinner: Spinach and Ricotta Stuffed Shells
- Snack: Veggie Sushi Rolls
- Dessert: Fruit Salad with Honey-Lime Dressing

Day 5:

- Breakfast: Greek Yogurt Parfait with Nuts and Fru
- Lunch: Quinoa Salad with Roasted Vegetables
- Dinner: Vegetable Curry with Quinoa
- Snack: Caprese Skewers
- Dessert: Apple Crisp with Almond Flour

Day 6:

- Breakfast: Tofu Scramble with Spinach
- Lunch: Stuffed Bell Peppers with Rice and Beans
- Dinner: Portobello Mushroom Burgers
- Snack: Edamame with Sea Salt

- Dessert: Greek Yogurt Berry Popsicles

Day 7:

- Breakfast: Whole Wheat Pancakes with Fruit Compote
- Lunch: Spinach and Strawberry Salad with Poppy Seed Dressing
- Dinner: Zucchini Noodles with Pesto
- Snack: Baked Sweet Potato Fries
- Dessert: Dark Chocolate Covered Strawberries

Week 2:

Day 8:

- Breakfast: Zucchini and Feta Frittata
- Lunch: Mediterranean Veggie Sandwich
- Dinner: Mexican Stuffed Peppers
- Snack: Cucumber and Cream Cheese Roll-Ups
- Dessert: Baked Apples with Cinnamon and Nutmeg

Day 9:

- Breakfast: Breakfast Burrito with Black Beans and Salsa

- Lunch: Sweet Potato and Black Bean Quesadilla

- Dinner: Lentil Shepherd's Pie

- Snack: Stuffed Mushrooms with Herbs and Cheese

- Dessert: Coconut Chia Seed Pudding

Day 10:

- Breakfast: Overnight Oats with Almond Milk and Nut Butter

- Lunch: Ratatouille with Couscous

- Dinner: Tofu Stir-Fry with Cashews

- Snack: Greek Yogurt Dip with Veggies

- Dessert: Pumpkin Pie Bites

Day 11:

- Breakfast: Spinach and Mushroom Breakfast Quesadilla

- Lunch: Thai Peanut Noodle Salad

- Dinner: Spinach and Artichoke Stuffed Spaghetti Squash

- Snack: Fruit and Cheese Platter

- Dessert: Almond Butter Cookies

Day 12:

- Breakfast: Veggie Breakfast Casserole
- Lunch: Greek Salad with Tofu Feta
- Dinner: Vegetarian Chili
- Snack: Avocado Bruschetta
- Dessert: Mango Sorbet

Day 13:

- Breakfast: Banana Walnut Muffins
- Lunch: Veggie Stir-Fry with Brown Rice
- Dinner: Mushroom and Spinach Lasagna
- Snack: Spinach and Artichoke Dip with Whole Wheat Pita
- Dessert: Carrot Cake Bites

Day 14:

- Breakfast: Veggie Breakfast Wrap
- Lunch: Tomato Basil Bruschetta
- Dinner: Thai Green Curry with Tofu
- Snack: Trail Mix with Nuts and Dried Fruit
- Dessert: Frozen Yogurt Bark with Berries

Week 3:

Day 15:

- Breakfast: Berry Smoothie Bowl
- Lunch: Lentil and Vegetable Soup
- Dinner: Cauliflower Rice Stir Fry
- Snack: Guacamole with Veggie Sticks
- Dessert: Berry Crisp with Oat Topping

Day 16:

- Breakfast: Avocado Toast with Chickpeas
- Lunch: Caprese Salad with Balsamic Glaze
- Dinner: Eggplant Parmesan
- Snack: Hummus and Whole Grain Crackers
- Dessert: Chocolate Avocado Mousse

Day 17:

- Breakfast: Vegetable Omelette
- Lunch: Chickpea Salad with Lemon Tahini Dressin
- Dinner: Butternut Squash Risotto
- Snack: Roasted Chickpeas
- Dessert: Banana Bread with Walnuts

Day 18:

- Breakfast: Chia Seed Pudding with Berries
- Lunch: Grilled Vegetable Wrap with Hummus
- Dinner: Spinach and Ricotta Stuffed Shells
- Snack: Veggie Sushi Rolls
- Dessert: Fruit Salad with Honey-Lime Dressing

Day 19:

- Breakfast: Greek Yogurt Parfait with Nuts and Fruit
- Lunch: Quinoa Salad with Roasted Vegetables
- Dinner: Vegetable Curry with Quinoa
- Snack: Caprese Skewers
- Dessert: Apple Crisp with Almond Flour

Day 20:

- Breakfast: Tofu Scramble with Spinach
- Lunch: Stuffed Bell Peppers with Rice and Beans
- Dinner: Portobello Mushroom Burgers
- Snack: Edamame with Sea Salt
- Dessert: Greek Yogurt Berry Popsicles

Day 21:

- Breakfast: Whole Wheat Pancakes with Fruit Compote
- Lunch: Spinach and Strawberry Salad with Poppy Seed Dressing
- Dinner: Zucchini Noodles with Pesto
- Snack: Baked Sweet Potato Fries
- Dessert: Dark Chocolate Covered Strawberries

Week 4:

Day 22:

- Breakfast: Zucchini and Feta Frittata
- Lunch: Mediterranean Veggie Sandwich
- Dinner: Mexican Stuffed Peppers
- Snack: Cucumber and Cream Cheese Roll-Ups
- Dessert: Baked Apples with Cinnamon and Nutmeg

Day 23:

- Breakfast: Breakfast Burrito with Black Beans and Salsa
- Lunch: Sweet Potato and Black Bean Quesadilla
- Dinner: Lentil Shepherd's Pie

- Snack: Stuffed Mushrooms with Herbs and Cheese

- Dessert: Coconut Chia Seed Pudding

Day 24:

- Breakfast: Overnight Oats with Almond Milk and Nut Butter

- Lunch: Ratatouille with Couscous

- Dinner: Tofu Stir-Fry with Cashews

- Snack: Greek Yogurt Dip with Veggies

- Dessert: Pumpkin Pie Bites

Day 25:

- Breakfast: Spinach and Mushroom Breakfast Quesadilla

- Lunch: Thai Peanut Noodle Salad

- Dinner: Spinach and Artichoke Stuffed Spaghetti Squash

- Snack: Fruit and Cheese Platter

- Dessert: Almond Butter Cookies

Day 26:

- Breakfast: Veggie Breakfast Casserole

- Lunch: Greek Salad with Tofu Feta

- Dinner: Vegetarian Chili

- Snack: Avocado Bruschetta

- Dessert: Mango Sorbet

Day 27:

- Breakfast: Banana Walnut Muffins

- Lunch: Veggie Stir-Fry with Brown Rice

- Dinner: Mushroom and Spinach Lasagna

- Snack: Spinach and Artichoke Dip with Whole Wheat Pita

- Dessert: Carrot Cake Bites

Day 28:

- Breakfast: Veggie Breakfast Wrap

- Lunch: Tomato Basil Bruschetta

- Dinner: Thai Green Curry with Tofu

- Snack: Trail Mix with Nuts and Dried Fruit

- Dessert: Frozen Yogurt Bark with Berries

Day 29:

- Breakfast: Berry Smoothie Bowl

- Lunch: Lentil and Vegetable Soup

- Dinner: Cauliflower Rice Stir Fry

- Snack: Guacamole with Veggie Sticks

- Dessert: Berry Crisp with Oat Topping

Day 30:

- Breakfast: Avocado Toast with Chickpeas

- Lunch: Caprese Salad with Balsamic Glaze

- Dinner: Eggplant Parmesan

- Snack: Hummus and Whole Grain Crackers

- Dessert: Chocolate Avocado Mousse

Chapter 2: Breakfast Recipes

These vegetarian breakfast recipes are specially crafted to provide you with the energy and nutrients you need to tackle your day while managing gestational diabetes. Each recipe is packed with flavor and wholesome ingredients to keep you satisfied and nourished.

Quinoa Breakfast Bowl

Ingredients:

- 1/2 cup cooked quinoa
- 1/4 cup sliced almonds
- 1/2 cup mixed berries
- 1 tablespoon honey
- 1/4 teaspoon cinnamon

Instructions:

1. In a bowl, combine cooked quinoa and sliced almonds.
2. Top with mixed berries.
3. Drizzle with honey and sprinkle with cinnamon.
4. Enjoy!

Nutrition Information:

- Calories: 320
- Protein: 10g
- Carbohydrates: 45g
- Fat: 12g
- Fiber: 6g
- Sugar: 15g
- Portion Size: 1 bowl

Avocado Toast with Chickpeas

Ingredients:

- 2 slices whole grain bread
- 1 ripe avocado
- 1/2 cup canned chickpeas, drained and rinsed
- Salt and pepper to taste
- Red pepper flakes (optional)

Instructions:

1. Toast the whole grain bread slices until golden brown.
2. Mash the ripe avocado and spread it evenly on the toast.

3. Top with chickpeas and season with salt, pepper, an

    red pepper flakes if desired.

4. Serve immediately.

Nutrition Information:

- Calories: 380

- Protein: 14g

- Carbohydrates: 40g

- Fat: 20g

- Fiber: 15g

- Sugar: 2g

- Portion Size: 1 serving (2 slices)

Vegetable Omelette

Ingredients:

- 2 eggs

- 1/4 cup chopped mixed vegetables (bell peppe
  onions, spinach, mushrooms)

- 1 tablespoon olive oil

- Salt and pepper to taste

- 2 tablespoons shredded cheese (optional)

Instructions:

1. In a bowl, beat the eggs and season with salt and pepper.
2. Heat olive oil in a non-stick skillet over medium heat.
3. Add the chopped vegetables and sauté until tender.
4. Pour the beaten eggs over the vegetables in the skillet.
5. Cook until the eggs are set, then sprinkle with shredded cheese if using.
6. Fold the omelette in half and serve hot.

Nutrition Information:

- Calories: 280
- Protein: 15g
- Carbohydrates: 6g
- Fat: 20g
- Fiber: 2g
- Sugar: 3g
- Portion Size: 1 omelette

Chia Seed Pudding with Berries

Ingredients:

- 2 tablespoons chia seeds
- 1/2 cup unsweetened almond milk
- 1/4 teaspoon vanilla extract
- 1/2 cup mixed berries
- 1 tablespoon honey or maple syrup (optional)

Instructions:

1. In a bowl, mix chia seeds, almond milk, and vanilla extract.
2. Let it sit for 10 minutes, stirring occasionally until thickened.
3. Top with mixed berries and drizzle with honey or maple syrup if desired.
4. Serve chilled.

Nutrition Information:

- Calories: 180
- Protein: 5g
- Carbohydrates: 20g
- Fat: 9g

- Fiber: 10g

- Sugar: 8g

- Portion Size: 1 serving

Greek Yogurt Parfait with Nuts and Fruit

Ingredients:

- 1/2 cup Greek yogurt

- 1/4 cup mixed nuts (almonds, walnuts, pecans)

- 1/2 cup mixed fruit (berries, sliced banana, kiwi)

- 1 tablespoon honey or maple syrup (optional)

Instructions:

1. In a glass or bowl, layer Greek yogurt, mixed nuts, and mixed fruit.

2. Drizzle with honey or maple syrup if desired.

3. Repeat layers if needed.

4. Serve immediately.

Nutrition Information:

- Calories: 280

- Protein: 15g

- Carbohydrates: 20g

- Fat: 15g

- Fiber: 5g

- Sugar: 12g

- Portion Size: 1 serving

Tofu Scramble with Spinach

Ingredients:

- 1/2 cup firm tofu, crumbled

- 1 cup fresh spinach leaves

- 1/4 cup diced tomatoes

- 1/4 teaspoon turmeric powder

- Salt and pepper to taste

- 1 teaspoon olive oil

Instructions:

1. Heat olive oil in a skillet over medium heat.

2. Add crumbled tofu and sauté for 2-3 minutes.

3. Add spinach and diced tomatoes, cook until spinach wilts.

4. Season with turmeric powder, salt, and pepper.

5. Serve hot.

Nutrition Information:

- Calories: 180
- Protein: 12g
- Carbohydrates: 8g
- Fat: 10g
- Fiber: 3g
- Sugar: 2g
- Portion Size: 1 serving

Whole Wheat Pancakes with Fruit Compote

Ingredients:

- 1 cup whole wheat flour
- 1 tablespoon baking powder
- 1 tablespoon honey or maple syrup
- 1 cup unsweetened almond milk
- 1 teaspoon vanilla extract
- Mixed fruit compote (berries, sliced peaches, etc.)

Instructions:

1. In a bowl, whisk together whole wheat flour an
    baking powder.
2. Add honey or maple syrup, almond milk, and vanil
    extract. Mix until smooth.
3. Heat a non-stick skillet over medium heat and light
    grease with oil.
4. Pour batter onto the skillet to form pancakes.
5. Cook until bubbles form on the surface, then flip ar
    cook until golden brown.
6. Serve with mixed fruit compote on top.

Nutrition Information:

- Calories: 220
- Protein: 6g
- Carbohydrates: 40g
- Fat: 4g
- Fiber: 6g
- Sugar: 12g
- Portion Size: 2 pancakes with fruit compote

Zucchini and Feta Frittata

Ingredients:

- 4 eggs
- 1 small zucchini, grated
- 1/4 cup crumbled feta cheese
- 1/4 cup chopped fresh herbs (parsley, basil)
- Salt and pepper to taste
- 1 teaspoon olive oil

Instructions:

1. Preheat the oven to 350°F (175°C).
2. In a bowl, beat the eggs and season with salt and pepper.
3. Stir in grated zucchini, crumbled feta cheese, and chopped herbs.
4. Heat olive oil in an oven-safe skillet over medium heat.
5. Pour the egg mixture into the skillet and cook for 2-3 minutes.
6. Transfer the skillet to the preheated oven and bake for 15-20 minutes, or until the frittata is set.
7. Slice and serve hot or cold.

Nutrition Information:

- Calories: 220
- Protein: 15g
- Carbohydrates: 6g
- Fat: 15g
- Fiber: 2g
- Sugar: 3g
- Portion Size: 1/4 of frittata

Breakfast Burrito with Black Beans and Salsa

Ingredients:

- 1 whole wheat tortilla
- 1/4 cup cooked black beans
- 2 eggs, scrambled
- 2 tablespoons salsa
- 2 tablespoons shredded cheese (optional)
- Salt and pepper to taste
- 1 teaspoon olive oil

Instructions:

1. Heat olive oil in a skillet over medium heat.
2. Warm the whole wheat tortilla in the skillet for about 30 seconds on each side.
3. Remove tortilla from the skillet and set aside.
4. In the same skillet, scramble the eggs until cooked through.
5. Spread the black beans, scrambled eggs, salsa, and shredded cheese (if using) in the center of the tortilla.
6. Season with salt and pepper.
7. Fold in the sides of the tortilla and roll it up into a burrito.
8. Serve hot.

Nutrition Information:

- Calories: 330
- Protein: 18g
- Carbohydrates: 30g
- Fat: 14g
- Fiber: 8g
- Sugar: 3g
- Portion Size: 1 burrito

Overnight Oats with Almond Milk and Nut Butter

Ingredients:

- 1/2 cup rolled oats
- 1/2 cup unsweetened almond milk
- 1 tablespoon nut butter (peanut butter, almond butter)
- 1 tablespoon chia seeds
- 1 tablespoon honey or maple syrup
- Mixed berries for topping

Instructions:

1. In a jar or bowl, combine rolled oats, almond milk, nut butter, chia seeds, and honey or maple syrup.
2. Stir well to combine.
3. Cover and refrigerate overnight.
4. In the morning, top with mixed berries before serving.

Nutrition Information:

- Calories: 350
- Protein: 12g

- Carbohydrates: 45g
- Fat: 15g
- Fiber: 9g
- Sugar: 10g
- Portion Size: 1 serving

Spinach and Mushroom Breakfast Quesadilla

Ingredients:

- 2 whole wheat tortillas
- 1 cup fresh spinach leaves
- 1/2 cup sliced mushrooms
- 1/4 cup shredded cheese (cheddar, mozzarella)
- Salt and pepper to taste
- 1 teaspoon olive oil

Instructions:

1. Heat olive oil in a skillet over medium heat.
2. Add spinach and mushrooms to the skillet and sauté until wilted.
3. Season with salt and pepper.

4. Remove spinach and mushrooms from the skillet and set aside.

5. Place one tortilla in the skillet and sprinkle half of the shredded cheese on top.

6. Add the sautéed spinach and mushrooms on one half of the tortilla.

7. Fold the other half of the tortilla over the filling.

8. Cook for 2-3 minutes on each side, until the tortilla is golden brown and the cheese is melted.

9. Repeat with the remaining tortilla and filling.

10. Cut each quesadilla into wedges and serve hot.

Nutrition Information:

- Calories: 280
- Protein: 12g
- Carbohydrates: 25g
- Fat: 15g
- Fiber: 5g
- Sugar: 2g
- Portion Size: 1 quesadilla

Veggie Breakfast Casserole

Ingredients:

- 6 eggs
- 1/2 cup milk (dairy or non-dairy)
- 1 cup diced vegetables (bell peppers, onions, broccoli)
- 1 cup shredded cheese (cheddar, Swiss)
- Salt and pepper to taste
- 1 teaspoon olive oil

Instructions:

1. Preheat the oven to 350°F (175°C) and grease a baking dish with olive oil.
2. In a bowl, whisk together eggs and milk. Season with salt and pepper.
3. Stir in diced vegetables and shredded cheese.
4. Pour the mixture into the prepared baking dish.
5. Bake for 25-30 minutes, or until the eggs are set and the top is golden brown.
6. Let cool slightly before slicing and serving.

Nutrition Information:

- Calories: 220
- Protein: 15g
- Carbohydrates: 8g
- Fat: 15g
- Fiber: 2g
- Sugar: 3g
- Portion Size: 1/6 of casserole

Banana Walnut Muffins

Ingredients:

- 1 cup whole wheat flour
- 1/2 cup rolled oats
- 1 teaspoon baking powder
- 1/2 teaspoon baking soda
- 1/4 teaspoon salt
- 2 ripe bananas, mashed
- 1/4 cup honey or maple syrup
- 1/4 cup unsweetened applesauce
- 1/4 cup chopped walnuts
- 1/4 cup unsweetened almond milk
- 1 teaspoon vanilla extract

nstructions:

1. Preheat the oven to 350°F (175°C) and line a muffin tin with paper liners.
2. In a bowl, whisk together whole wheat flour, rolled oats, baking powder, baking soda, and salt.
3. In another bowl, mix mashed bananas, honey or maple syrup, applesauce, almond milk, and vanilla extract.
4. Combine the wet and dry ingredients, then fold in the chopped walnuts.
5. Divide the batter evenly among the muffin cups.
6. Bake for 18-20 minutes, or until a toothpick inserted into the center comes out clean.
7. Let cool in the muffin tin for 5 minutes, then transfer to a wire rack to cool completely.

Nutrition Information:

- Calories: 160
- Protein: 4g
- Carbohydrates: 28g
- Fat: 5g
- Fiber: 3g

- Sugar: 12g

- Portion Size: 1 muffin

Veggie Breakfast Wrap

Ingredients:

- 1 whole wheat tortilla

- 2 eggs, scrambled

- 1/4 cup diced bell peppers

- 1/4 cup diced onions

- 1/4 cup diced tomatoes

- 1/4 cup shredded cheese (cheddar, pepper jack)

- Salt and pepper to taste

- Salsa or hot sauce for serving (optional)

Instructions:

1. Heat a non-stick skillet over medium heat.

2. Add diced bell peppers and onions to the skillet an
   sauté until softened.

3. Push the vegetables to one side of the skillet and ad
   the scrambled eggs to the other side.

4. Cook the eggs until set, then combine with th
   vegetables.

5. Warm the whole wheat tortilla in the skillet for about 30 seconds on each side.

6. Place the scrambled eggs and vegetables in the center of the tortilla.

7. Top with diced tomatoes and shredded cheese.

8. Season with salt and pepper.

9. Fold in the sides of the tortilla and roll it up into a wrap.

10. Serve with salsa or hot sauce if desired.

Nutrition Information:

- Calories: 300
- Protein: 15g
- Carbohydrates: 20g
- Fat: 15g
- Fiber: 3g
- Sugar: 3g
- Portion Size: 1 wrap

Berry Smoothie Bowl

Ingredients:

- 1 frozen banana

- 1/2 cup mixed berries (strawberries, blueberries, raspberries)
- 1/2 cup unsweetened almond milk
- 1 tablespoon chia seeds
- Toppings: sliced fresh fruit, granola, shredded coconut, nuts, seeds

Instructions:

1. In a blender, combine the frozen banana, mixed berries, almond milk, and chia seeds.
2. Blend until smooth and creamy, adding more almond milk if needed to reach desired consistency.
3. Pour the smoothie into a bowl.
4. Top with sliced fresh fruit, granola, shredded coconut, nuts, and seeds.
5. Serve immediately with a spoon.

Nutrition Information:

- Calories: 280
- Protein: 5g
- Carbohydrates: 45g
- Fat: 10g

- Fiber: 12g
- Sugar: 20g
- Portion Size: 1 bowl

Chapter 3: Lunch Recipes

In this chapter, we present a diverse array of lunch recipes designed to tantalize your taste buds while providing essential nutrients to support your health. From hearty soups to vibrant salads and filling wraps, each recipe is crafted with a balance of flavors and textures to keep you energized throughout the day.

Lentil and Vegetable Soup

Ingredients:

- 1 cup lentils
- 2 carrots, diced
- 2 stalks celery, diced
- 1 onion, diced
- 3 cloves garlic, minced
- 6 cups vegetable broth
- 1 can diced tomatoes
- 1 teaspoon cumin
- Salt and pepper to taste
- Fresh parsley for garnish

1. In a large pot, sauté the onion and garlic until fragrant.
2. Add the carrots, celery, lentils, vegetable broth, diced tomatoes, and cumin to the pot.
3. Bring to a boil, then reduce heat and simmer for 20-25 minutes until lentils are tender.
4. Season with salt and pepper to taste.
5. Serve hot, garnished with fresh parsley.

Nutrition Information (per serving):

- Calories: 250
- Protein: 15g
- Carbohydrates: 45g
- Fat: 1g
- Fiber: 15g
- Sugar: 6g
- Portion Size: 1 cup

Caprese Salad with Balsamic Glaze

Ingredients:

- 2 ripe tomatoes, sliced

- 1 ball fresh mozzarella, sliced

- Fresh basil leaves

- Balsamic glaze

- Salt and pepper to taste

Instructions:

1. Arrange the tomato and mozzarella slices on a plate alternating with fresh basil leaves.

2. Drizzle with balsamic glaze.

3. Season with salt and pepper to taste.

4. Serve immediately.

Nutrition Information (per serving):

- Calories: 200

- Protein: 12g

- Carbohydrates: 8g

- Fat: 14g

- Fiber: 2g

- Sugar: 5g

- Portion Size: 1 salad

Chickpea Salad with Lemon Tahini Dressing

Ingredients:

- 1 can chickpeas, rinsed and drained
- 1 cucumber, diced
- 1 bell pepper, diced
- 1/4 cup red onion, diced
- 1/4 cup fresh parsley, chopped
- 2 tablespoons tahini
- 2 tablespoons lemon juice
- 1 tablespoon olive oil
- Salt and pepper to taste

Instructions:

1. In a large bowl, combine the chickpeas, cucumber, bell pepper, red onion, and parsley.
2. In a small bowl, whisk together the tahini, lemon juice, olive oil, salt, and pepper.
3. Pour the dressing over the salad and toss to coat evenly.
4. Serve chilled or at room temperature.

Nutrition Information (per serving):

- Calories: 280
- Protein: 9g
- Carbohydrates: 28g
- Fat: 16g
- Fiber: 7g
- Sugar: 6g
- Portion Size: 1 cup

Grilled Vegetable Wrap with Hummus

Ingredients:

- 1 zucchini, sliced
- 1 yellow squash, sliced
- 1 red bell pepper, sliced
- 1/2 red onion, sliced
- 4 whole wheat wraps
- 1/2 cup hummus
- Fresh spinach leaves
- Salt and pepper to taste

Instructions:

1. Preheat grill to medium-high heat.
2. Season the sliced vegetables with salt and pepper.
3. Grill the vegetables until tender and slightly charred, about 5-7 minutes per side.
4. Warm the wraps on the grill for 1-2 minutes.
5. Spread a layer of hummus onto each wrap.
6. Place grilled vegetables and fresh spinach leaves on top of the hummus.
7. Roll up the wraps tightly, securing with toothpicks if necessary.
8. Slice in half and serve.

Nutrition Information (per serving):

- Calories: 280
- Protein: 9g
- Carbohydrates: 45g
- Fat: 7g
- Fiber: 9g
- Sugar: 5g
- Portion Size: 1 wrap

Quinoa Salad with Roasted Vegetables

Ingredients:

- 1 cup quinoa, cooked
- 1 small eggplant, diced
- 1 zucchini, diced
- 1 red bell pepper, diced
- 1/4 cup cherry tomatoes, halved
- 2 tablespoons olive oil
- 1 tablespoon balsamic vinegar
- Salt and pepper to taste
- Fresh basil leaves for garnish

Instructions:

1. Preheat oven to 400°F (200°C).
2. In a large bowl, toss the diced eggplant, zucchini, red bell pepper, and cherry tomatoes with olive oil, balsamic vinegar, salt, and pepper.
3. Spread the vegetables in a single layer on a baking sheet.
4. Roast in the preheated oven for 20-25 minutes until vegetables are tender and slightly caramelized.

5. In a serving bowl, combine the cooked quinoa and roasted vegetables.

6. Garnish with fresh basil leaves before serving.

Nutrition Information (per serving):

- Calories: 320
- Protein: 8g
- Carbohydrates: 50g
- Fat: 10g
- Fiber: 9g
- Sugar: 6g
- Portion Size: 1 cup

Stuffed Bell Peppers with Rice and Beans

Ingredients:

- 4 bell peppers, halved and seeds removed
- 1 cup cooked brown rice
- 1 can black beans, rinsed and drained
- 1/2 cup corn kernels
- 1/2 cup diced tomatoes

- 1/4 cup chopped cilantro

- 1 teaspoon cumin

- 1/2 teaspoon chili powder

- Salt and pepper to taste

- 1/2 cup shredded cheese (optional)

Instructions:

1. Preheat oven to 375°F (190°C).

2. In a large bowl, mix together the cooked brown rice, black beans, corn kernels, diced tomatoes, cilantro, cumin, chili powder, salt, and pepper.

3. Stuff each bell pepper half with the rice and bean mixture.

4. Place stuffed peppers in a baking dish, and cover with aluminum foil.

5. Bake in the preheated oven for 25-30 minutes until peppers are tender.

6. If desired, sprinkle shredded cheese over the stuffed peppers during the last 5 minutes of baking.

7. Serve hot.

utrition Information (per serving):

- Calories: 280
- Protein: 12g
- Carbohydrates: 45g
- Fat: 6g
- Fiber: 10g
- Sugar: 6g
- Portion Size: 1 stuffed pepper half

pinach and Strawberry Salad with oppy Seed Dressing

gredients:

- 4 cups fresh spinach leaves
- 1 cup sliced strawberries
- 1/4 cup sliced almonds
- 2 tablespoons feta cheese, crumbled
- 2 tablespoons poppy seed dressing

structions:

1. In a large bowl, combine the fresh spinach leaves, sliced strawberries, sliced almonds, and crumbled feta cheese.

2. Drizzle with poppy seed dressing and toss gently
    coat.

3. Serve immediately.

Nutrition Information (per serving):

- Calories: 180
- Protein: 5g
- Carbohydrates: 15g
- Fat: 12g
- Fiber: 4g
- Sugar: 7g
- Portion Size: 2 cups

Mediterranean Veggie Sandwich

Ingredients:

- 4 whole wheat sandwich thins or bread slices
- 1/2 cup hummus
- 1/2 cup sliced cucumber
- 1/2 cup sliced bell peppers
- 1/4 cup sliced red onion
- 1/4 cup sliced black olives
- 1/4 cup crumbled feta cheese

- Fresh spinach leaves

Instructions:

1. Spread hummus on each sandwich thin or bread slice.
2. Layer cucumber slices, bell pepper slices, red onion slices, black olives, crumbled feta cheese, and fresh spinach leaves on one side of the sandwich.
3. Top with the other sandwich thin or bread slice to form a sandwich.
4. Slice in half and serve.

Nutrition Information (per serving):

- Calories: 280
- Protein: 10g
- Carbohydrates: 35g
- Fat: 12g
- Fiber: 8g
- Sugar: 6g
- Portion Size: 1 sandwich

Sweet Potato and Black Bean Quesadilla

Ingredients:

- 2 medium sweet potatoes, cooked and mashed
- 1 can black beans, rinsed and drained
- 1 teaspoon chili powder
- 1/2 teaspoon cumin
- 4 whole wheat tortillas
- 1 cup shredded cheese (optional)
- Fresh cilantro for garnish
- Salsa and Greek yogurt for serving (optional)

Instructions:

1. In a bowl, mix together the mashed sweet potatoes, black beans, chili powder, and cumin.
2. Spread the sweet potato and black bean mixture evenly onto two tortillas.
3. Sprinkle shredded cheese on top if desired, then cover each with another tortilla.
4. Heat a non-stick skillet over medium heat.
5. Cook each quesadilla for 2-3 minutes on each side until golden brown and crispy.

6. Slice into wedges and garnish with fresh cilantro.

7. Serve with salsa and Greek yogurt if desired.

Nutrition Information (per serving):

- Calories: 320
- Protein: 12g
- Carbohydrates: 45g
- Fat: 10g
- Fiber: 8g
- Sugar: 5g
- Portion Size: 1 quesadilla

Ratatouille with Couscous

Ingredients:

- 1 eggplant, diced
- 2 zucchinis, diced
- 1 bell pepper, diced
- 1 onion, diced
- 2 cloves garlic, minced
- 1 can diced tomatoes
- 1 teaspoon dried thyme
- 1 teaspoon dried oregano

- Salt and pepper to taste
- 1 cup couscous, cooked
- Fresh basil for garnish

Instructions:

1. In a large skillet, sauté the diced eggplant, zucchini, bell pepper, onion, and garlic until softened.
2. Add the diced tomatoes, dried thyme, dried oregano, salt, and pepper to the skillet. Stir to combine.
3. Simmer the mixture for 15-20 minutes until vegetables are tender and flavors are well combined.
4. Serve the ratatouille over cooked couscous.
5. Garnish with fresh basil before serving.

Nutrition Information (per serving):

- Calories: 280
- Protein: 8g
- Carbohydrates: 55g
- Fat: 2g
- Fiber: 10g
- Sugar: 8g
- Portion Size: 1 cup ratatouille with 1/2 cup couscous

hai Peanut Noodle Salad

gredients:

- 8 oz rice noodles, cooked and cooled
- 1 cup shredded cabbage
- 1 carrot, julienned
- 1/2 cucumber, thinly sliced
- 1/4 cup chopped peanuts
- 1/4 cup chopped cilantro
- 1/4 cup sliced green onions
- 1/4 cup peanut butter
- 2 tablespoons soy sauce
- 2 tablespoons lime juice
- 1 tablespoon honey
- 1 teaspoon sriracha (optional)
- 1 clove garlic, minced

structions:

1. In a large bowl, combine the cooked rice noodles, shredded cabbage, julienned carrot, sliced cucumber, chopped peanuts, chopped cilantro, and sliced green onions.

2. In a small bowl, whisk together the peanut butter, s
   sauce, lime juice, honey, sriracha (if using), a
   minced garlic to make the dressing.

3. Pour the dressing over the noodle salad and toss
   coat evenly.

4. Serve chilled or at room temperature.

Nutrition Information (per serving):

- Calories: 320
- Protein: 10g
- Carbohydrates: 45g
- Fat: 12g
- Fiber: 6g
- Sugar: 8g
- Portion Size: 1.5 cups

Greek Salad with Tofu Feta

Ingredients:

- 4 cups chopped romaine lettuce
- 1 cucumber, diced
- 1 bell pepper, diced
- 1 cup cherry tomatoes, halved

- 1/4 cup sliced red onion
- 1/4 cup kalamata olives
- 1/4 cup crumbled tofu feta
- 2 tablespoons olive oil
- 2 tablespoons red wine vinegar
- 1 teaspoon dried oregano
- Salt and pepper to taste

Instructions:

1. In a large bowl, combine the chopped romaine lettuce, diced cucumber, diced bell pepper, cherry tomatoes, sliced red onion, kalamata olives, and crumbled tofu feta.
2. In a small bowl, whisk together the olive oil, red wine vinegar, dried oregano, salt, and pepper to make the dressing.
3. Pour the dressing over the salad and toss to coat evenly.
4. Serve immediately.

Nutrition Information (per serving):
- Calories: 200

- Protein: 8g

- Carbohydrates: 15g

- Fat: 12g

- Fiber: 6g

- Sugar: 5g

- Portion Size: 2 cups

Veggie Stir-Fry with Brown Rice

Ingredients:

- 1 cup brown rice, cooked

- 1 tablespoon sesame oil

- 2 cups mixed vegetables (such as bell peppers, broccoli, carrots, snap peas)

- 2 cloves garlic, minced

- 1 tablespoon soy sauce

- 1 tablespoon hoisin sauce

- 1 teaspoon sriracha (optional)

- 2 green onions, sliced

- Sesame seeds for garnish

1. Heat sesame oil in a large skillet or wok over medium-high heat.
2. Add mixed vegetables and minced garlic to the skillet. Stir-fry for 3-4 minutes until vegetables are tender-crisp.
3. In a small bowl, whisk together soy sauce, hoisin sauce, and sriracha (if using).
4. Pour the sauce over the vegetables and stir to coat evenly.
5. Add cooked brown rice to the skillet and toss to combine.
6. Cook for an additional 2-3 minutes until heated through.
7. Garnish with sliced green onions and sesame seeds before serving.

Nutrition Information (per serving):

- Calories: 300
- Protein: 8g
- Carbohydrates: 50g
- Fat: 8g

- Fiber: 8g
- Sugar: 5g
- Portion Size: 1 cup stir-fry with 1/2 cup brown rice

Tomato Basil Bruschetta

Ingredients:

- 4 slices whole wheat baguette
- 2 tomatoes, diced
- 2 tablespoons chopped fresh basil
- 1 clove garlic, minced
- 1 tablespoon balsamic vinegar
- 1 tablespoon olive oil
- Salt and pepper to taste

Instructions:

1. Preheat oven to 400°F (200°C).
2. Place whole wheat baguette slices on a baking sheet and toast in the preheated oven for 5-7 minutes until crispy.
3. In a bowl, combine diced tomatoes, chopped fresh basil, minced garlic, balsamic vinegar, olive oil, salt and pepper.

4. Spoon the tomato mixture onto the toasted baguette slices.

5. Serve immediately.

Nutrition Information (per serving):

- Calories: 120
- Protein: 3g
- Carbohydrates: 18g
- Fat: 4g
- Fiber: 3g
- Sugar: 3g
- Portion Size: 2 slices

Spinach and Goat Cheese Stuffed Portobello Mushrooms

Ingredients:

- 4 large portobello mushrooms, stems removed
- 2 cups fresh spinach leaves
- 1/2 cup crumbled goat cheese
- 2 cloves garlic, minced
- 2 tablespoons olive oil

- Salt and pepper to taste

Instructions:

1. Preheat oven to 375°F (190°C).
2. Brush portobello mushrooms with olive oil and season with salt and pepper.
3. In a skillet, sauté fresh spinach leaves and minced garlic until wilted.
4. Fill each portobello mushroom cap with sautéed spinach and crumbled goat cheese.
5. Place stuffed mushrooms on a baking sheet and bake in the preheated oven for 15-20 minutes until mushrooms are tender and cheese is melted.
6. Serve hot.

Nutrition Information (per serving):

- Calories: 150
- Protein: 8g
- Carbohydrates: 5g
- Fat: 10g
- Fiber: 2g
- Sugar: 2g
- Portion Size: 1 stuffed mushroom

Chapter 4: Dinner Recipes

These recipes are designed to cater to vegetarians managing gestational diabetes, providing a variety of flavors and textures to keep your meals exciting and enjoyable. From hearty casseroles to flavorful stir-fries, each recipe offers a balance of essential nutrients while keeping carbohydrate content in check.

Cauliflower Rice Stir Fry

Ingredients:

- 1 head cauliflower, grated into rice
- 2 cups mixed vegetables (bell peppers, broccoli, carrots)
- 1 cup tofu, cubed
- 2 cloves garlic, minced
- 2 tablespoons soy sauce
- 1 tablespoon sesame oil
- Salt and pepper to taste

Instructions:

1. In a large skillet, heat sesame oil over medium heat. Add minced garlic and cook until fragrant.
2. Add cubed tofu to the skillet and cook until lightly browned.
3. Add mixed vegetables and cauliflower rice to the skillet. Cook until vegetables are tender.
4. Stir in soy sauce and season with salt and pepper to taste.
5. Serve hot.

Nutrition Information:

- Calories: 250
- Protein: 15g
- Carbohydrates: 20g
- Fat: 12g
- Fiber: 8g
- Sugar: 6g
- Portion Size: 1 ½ cups

Eggplant Parmesan

Ingredients:

- 2 large eggplants, sliced into rounds
- 1 cup whole wheat breadcrumbs
- 1 cup grated Parmesan cheese
- 2 cups marinara sauce
- 1 cup shredded mozzarella cheese
- 2 tablespoons olive oil
- Salt and pepper to taste

Instructions:

1. Prcheat oven to 375°F (190°C).
2. Dip eggplant slices in olive oil, then coat with breadcrumbs mixed with Parmesan cheese.
3. Place coated eggplant slices on a baking sheet and bake for 20-25 minutes, or until golden brown.
4. In a baking dish, spread a layer of marinara sauce. Place baked eggplant slices on top, then cover with remaining marinara sauce.
5. Sprinkle shredded mozzarella cheese on top.
6. Bake for an additional 15-20 minutes, or until cheese is melted and bubbly.
7. Serve hot.

Nutrition Information:

- Calories: 320
- Protein: 15g
- Carbohydrates: 25g
- Fat: 18g
- Fiber: 7g
- Sugar: 10g
- Portion Size: 2 slices

Butternut Squash Risotto

Ingredients:

- 1 butternut squash, peeled and diced
- 1 ½ cups Arborio rice
- 4 cups vegetable broth
- 1 onion, diced
- 2 cloves garlic, minced
- ½ cup grated Parmesan cheese
- 2 tablespoons olive oil
- Salt and pepper to taste

structions:

1. In a large pot, heat olive oil over medium heat. Add diced onion and garlic, and cook until softened.

2. Add Arborio rice to the pot and cook for 1-2 minutes, stirring constantly.

3. Gradually add vegetable broth, 1 cup at a time, stirring frequently and allowing the rice to absorb the liquid before adding more.

4. Once the rice is almost tender, stir in diced butternut squash and continue cooking until the squash is tender and the risotto is creamy.

5. Remove from heat and stir in grated Parmesan cheese. Season with salt and pepper to taste.

6. Serve hot.

utrition Information:

- Calories: 280
- Protein: 7g
- Carbohydrates: 45g
- Fat: 8g
- Fiber: 5g
- Sugar: 3g
- Portion Size: 1 cup

Spinach and Ricotta Stuffed Shells

Ingredients:

- 16 jumbo pasta shells
- 2 cups fresh spinach, chopped
- 1 cup ricotta cheese
- 1 cup marinara sauce
- ½ cup shredded mozzarella cheese
- 2 tablespoons grated Parmesan cheese
- 1 teaspoon dried Italian seasoning
- Salt and pepper to taste

Instructions:

1. Preheat oven to 375°F (190°C). Cook pasta she
   according to package instructions, then drain and s
   aside.
2. In a mixing bowl, combine chopped spinach, rico
   cheese, dried Italian seasoning, salt, and pepper.
3. Stuff each cooked pasta shell with the spinach a
   ricotta mixture.
4. Spread a thin layer of marinara sauce on the bott
   of a baking dish. Place stuffed shells in the dish.

5. Top stuffed shells with remaining marinara sauce and sprinkle with shredded mozzarella and grated Parmesan cheese.

6. Cover the baking dish with foil and bake for 20 minutes. Remove foil and bake for an additional 10 minutes, or until cheese is melted and bubbly.

7. Serve hot.

Nutrition Information:

- Calories: 310
- Protein: 15g
- Carbohydrates: 35g
- Fat: 12g
- Fiber: 5g
- Sugar: 5g
- Portion Size: 4 shells

Vegetable Curry with Quinoa

Ingredients:

- 1 cup quinoa, rinsed
- 2 cups mixed vegetables (bell peppers, carrots, broccoli, peas)

- 1 can (14 oz) coconut milk
- 2 tablespoons curry powder
- 1 tablespoon olive oil
- Salt and pepper to taste
- Fresh cilantro for garnish (optional)

Instructions:

1. Cook quinoa according to package instructions and set aside.
2. In a large skillet, heat olive oil over medium heat. Add mixed vegetables and cook until tender.
3. Stir in curry powder and cook for an additional minute.
4. Pour in coconut milk and simmer for 5-7 minutes, or until the sauce thickens.
5. Season with salt and pepper to taste.
6. Serve vegetable curry over cooked quinoa, garnished with fresh cilantro if desired.

Nutrition Information:

- Calories: 320
- Protein: 8g

- Carbohydrates: 30g
- Fat: 20g
- Fiber: 6g
- Sugar: 3g
- Portion Size: 1 cup curry with ½ cup quinoa

Portobello Mushroom Burgers

Ingredients:

- 4 large portobello mushroom caps
- 4 whole wheat burger buns
- 1 avocado, sliced
- 1 tomato, sliced
- 1 cup arugula
- ¼ cup balsamic vinegar
- 2 tablespoons olive oil
- Salt and pepper to taste

Instructions:

1. Preheat grill or grill pan over medium heat.
2. In a small bowl, whisk together balsamic vinegar, olive oil, salt, and pepper.

3. Brush mushroom caps with the balsamic mixture and place on the grill.

4. Grill mushrooms for 4-5 minutes on each side, or until tender.

5. Toast burger buns on the grill for 1-2 minutes.

6. Assemble burgers by placing grilled mushroom caps on the bottom half of each bun.

7. Top with sliced avocado, tomato, and arugula. Cover with the top half of the bun.

8. Serve hot.

Nutrition Information:

- Calories: 280
- Protein: 10g
- Carbohydrates: 35g
- Fat: 12g
- Fiber: 8g
- Sugar: 6g
- Portion Size: 1 burger

ucchini Noodles with Pesto

gredients:

- 4 medium zucchinis, spiralized into noodles
- 1 cup fresh basil leaves
- ⅓ cup pine nuts
- 2 cloves garlic
- ¼ cup grated Parmesan cheese
- ¼ cup olive oil
- Salt and pepper to taste
- Cherry tomatoes for garnish (optional)

structions:

1. In a food processor, combine basil leaves, pine nuts, garlic, and Parmesan cheese. Pulse until finely chopped.
2. With the food processor running, slowly drizzle in olive oil until pesto is smooth.
3. Heat a large skillet over medium heat. Add zucchini noodles and cook for 2-3 minutes, or until just tender.
4. Stir in pesto sauce and toss to coat the noodles evenly.
5. Season with salt and pepper to taste.

6. Garnish with cherry tomatoes if desired befo
   serving.

Nutrition Information:

- Calories: 220
- Protein: 5g
- Carbohydrates: 10g
- Fat: 18g
- Fiber: 4g
- Sugar: 4g
- Portion Size: 1 ½ cups

Mexican Stuffed Peppers

Ingredients:

- 4 bell peppers, halved and seeds removed
- 1 cup cooked brown rice
- 1 cup black beans, drained and rinsed
- 1 cup corn kernels
- 1 cup salsa
- 1 cup shredded cheddar cheese
- 1 teaspoon chili powder
- 1 teaspoon cumin

- Salt and pepper to taste

- Fresh cilantro for garnish (optional)

Instructions:

1. Preheat oven to 375°F (190°C).

2. In a large mixing bowl, combine cooked brown rice, black beans, corn kernels, salsa, shredded cheddar cheese, chili powder, cumin, salt, and pepper.

3. Stuff each bell pepper half with the rice and bean mixture.

4. Place stuffed peppers in a baking dish and cover with foil.

5. Bake for 30 minutes.

6. Remove foil and bake for an additional 10 minutes, or until peppers are tender and cheese is melted.

7. Garnish with fresh cilantro before serving.

Nutrition Information:

- Calories: 280

- Protein: 15g

- Carbohydrates: 30g

- Fat: 12g

- Fiber: 8g

- Sugar: 6g

- Portion Size: 2 pepper halves

Lentil Shepherd's Pie

Ingredients:

- 2 cups cooked lentils

- 2 cups mixed vegetables (carrots, peas, corn)

- 1 onion, diced

- 2 cloves garlic, minced

- 1 cup vegetable broth

- 2 tablespoons tomato paste

- 2 tablespoons olive oil

- 4 cups mashed potatoes

- Salt and pepper to taste

- Fresh parsley for garnish (optional)

Instructions:

1. Preheat oven to 375°F (190°C).

2. In a large skillet, heat olive oil over medium heat. Add diced onion and minced garlic, and cook until softened.

3. Add mixed vegetables and cooked lentils to the skillet. Stir in vegetable broth and tomato paste. Cook for 5-7 minutes, or until vegetables are tender and mixture thickens.

4. Season with salt and pepper to taste.

5. Transfer lentil and vegetable mixture to a baking dish.

6. Spread mashed potatoes evenly over the lentil mixture.

7. Bake for 25-30 minutes, or until the top is golden brown.

8. Garnish with fresh parsley before serving.

Nutrition Information:

- Calories: 320
- Protein: 10g
- Carbohydrates: 45g
- Fat: 10g
- Fiber: 8g
- Sugar: 5g
- Portion Size: 1 cup

Tofu Stir-Fry with Cashews

Ingredients:

- 1 block tofu, pressed and cubed
- 2 cups mixed vegetables (bell peppers, broccoli, snap peas)
- ½ cup cashews
- 2 tablespoons soy sauce
- 1 tablespoon hoisin sauce
- 1 tablespoon sesame oil
- 2 cloves garlic, minced
- 1 teaspoon ginger, minced
- Salt and pepper to taste
- Cooked brown rice for serving

Instructions:

1. In a large skillet or wok, heat sesame oil over medium heat. Add minced garlic and ginger, and cook until fragrant.

2. Add cubed tofu to the skillet and cook until lightly browned on all sides.

3. Add mixed vegetables and cashews to the skillet. Stir-fry until vegetables are tender-crisp.

4. Stir in soy sauce and hoisin sauce, and cook for an additional 2-3 minutes.

5. Season with salt and pepper to taste.

6. Serve tofu stir-fry over cooked brown rice.

Nutrition Information:

- Calories: 350
- Protein: 15g
- Carbohydrates: 30g
- Fat: 20g
- Fiber: 6g
- Sugar: 5g
- Portion Size: 1 ½ cups stir-fry with ½ cup rice

Spinach and Artichoke Stuffed Spaghetti Squash

Ingredients:

- 2 spaghetti squash, halved and seeds removed
- 2 cups fresh spinach, chopped
- 1 can (14 oz) artichoke hearts, drained and chopped
- 1 cup ricotta cheese

- ½ cup grated Parmesan cheese
- 2 cloves garlic, minced
- 2 tablespoons olive oil
- Salt and pepper to taste

Instructions:

1. Preheat oven to 400°F (200°C).
2. Drizzle olive oil over the cut sides of the spaghe[tti] squash halves and season with salt and pepper.
3. Place squash halves cut-side down on a baking she[et] and bake for 30-40 minutes, or until tender.
4. In a skillet, heat olive oil over medium heat. A[dd] minced garlic and cook until fragrant.
5. Add chopped spinach and cook until wilted.
6. Stir in chopped artichoke hearts, ricotta cheese, a[nd] grated Parmesan cheese. Cook until heated throug[h].
7. Once spaghetti squash is done, use a fork to scra[pe] the flesh into strands.
8. Divide the spinach and artichoke mixture among t[he] spaghetti squash halves.
9. Return stuffed squash to the oven and bake for additional 10 minutes.
10. Serve hot.

Nutrition Information:

- Calories: 280
- Protein: 12g
- Carbohydrates: 20g
- Fat: 18g
- Fiber: 8g
- Sugar: 6g
- Portion Size: 1 stuffed squash half

Vegetarian Chili

Ingredients:

- 2 cans (14 oz each) diced tomatoes
- 1 can (15 oz) black beans, drained and rinsed
- 1 can (15 oz) kidney beans, drained and rinsed
- 1 cup corn kernels
- 1 onion, diced
- 2 cloves garlic, minced
- 1 bell pepper, diced
- 1 tablespoon chili powder
- 1 teaspoon cumin
- Salt and pepper to taste
- Fresh cilantro for garnish (optional)

Instructions:

1. In a large pot, heat olive oil over medium heat. Add diced onion, minced garlic, and diced bell pepper. Cook until softened.
2. Stir in chili powder and cumin, and cook for an additional minute.
3. Add diced tomatoes, black beans, kidney beans, and corn kernels to the pot. Stir to combine.
4. Bring chili to a simmer and let it cook for 20-25 minutes, stirring occasionally.
5. Season with salt and pepper to taste.
6. Serve hot, garnished with fresh cilantro if desired.

Nutrition Information:

- Calories: 250
- Protein: 10g
- Carbohydrates: 45g
- Fat: 2g
- Fiber: 12g
- Sugar: 8g
- Portion Size: 1 cup

Mushroom and Spinach Lasagna

Ingredients:

- 9 lasagna noodles, cooked according to package instructions
- 2 cups sliced mushrooms
- 2 cups fresh spinach
- 2 cups marinara sauce
- 1 cup ricotta cheese
- 1 cup shredded mozzarella cheese
- ½ cup grated Parmesan cheese
- 2 cloves garlic, minced
- 1 tablespoon olive oil
- Salt and pepper to taste

Instructions:

1. Preheat oven to 375°F (190°C).
2. In a skillet, heat olive oil over medium heat. Add minced garlic and cook until fragrant.
3. Add sliced mushrooms to the skillet and cook until tender.
4. Stir in fresh spinach and cook until wilted.

5. Spread a thin layer of marinara sauce on the bottom of a baking dish.

6. Layer cooked lasagna noodles on top of the sauce.

7. Spread half of the mushroom and spinach mixture over the noodles, then dollop half of the ricotta cheese on top.

8. Repeat the layers with marinara sauce, noodles, remaining mushroom and spinach mixture, and remaining ricotta cheese.

9. Top with shredded mozzarella and grated Parmesan cheese.

10. Cover with foil and bake for 30 minutes. Remove foil and bake for an additional 10 minutes, or until cheese is bubbly and golden.

11. Let lasagna cool for a few minutes before serving.

Nutrition Information:
- Calories: 350
- Protein: 18g
- Carbohydrates: 35g
- Fat: 15g
- Fiber: 5g

- Sugar: 8g
- Portion Size: 1/6 of lasagna

hai Green Curry with Tofu

gredients:

- 1 block tofu, cubed
- 2 cups mixed vegetables (bell peppers, broccoli, snap peas)
- 1 can (14 oz) coconut milk
- 3 tablespoons Thai green curry paste
- 2 tablespoons soy sauce
- 1 tablespoon brown sugar
- 1 tablespoon lime juice
- 2 tablespoons olive oil
- Fresh cilantro for garnish (optional)
- Cooked brown rice for serving

structions:

1. In a large skillet or wok, heat olive oil over medium heat. Add cubed tofu and cook until lightly browned on all sides. Remove tofu from the skillet and set aside.

2. In the same skillet, add mixed vegetables and coo[k]
    until tender-crisp.

3. Stir in Thai green curry paste and cook for 1
    minutes, until fragrant.

4. Pour in coconut milk, soy sauce, brown sugar, a[nd]
    lime juice. Stir to combine.

5. Add cooked tofu back to the skillet and simmer f[or]
    5-7 minutes, or until heated through and flavors a[re]
    blended.

6. Serve Thai green curry over cooked brown ri[ce]
    garnished with fresh cilantro if desired.

Nutrition Information:

- Calories: 380
- Protein: 15g
- Carbohydrates: 25g
- Fat: 25g
- Fiber: 5g
- Sugar: 6g
- Portion Size: 1 cup curry with ½ cup rice

Veggie Pizza with Whole Wheat Crust

Ingredients:

- 1 batch whole wheat pizza dough (store-bought or homemade)
- 1 cup marinara sauce
- 2 cups mixed vegetables (bell peppers, onions, mushrooms, spinach)
- 1 cup shredded mozzarella cheese
- ½ cup sliced black olives
- 1 tablespoon olive oil
- Salt and pepper to taste
- Fresh basil for garnish (optional)

Instructions:

1. Preheat oven to 450°F (230°C). If using a pizza stone, place it in the oven to preheat.
2. Roll out the pizza dough on a floured surface to your desired thickness.
3. Transfer the rolled-out dough to a pizza pan or parchment paper-lined baking sheet.

4. Spread marinara sauce evenly over the pizza dough, leaving a small border around the edges.

5. Arrange mixed vegetables and black olives over the sauce.

6. Sprinkle shredded mozzarella cheese on top of the vegetables.

7. Drizzle olive oil over the pizza and season with salt and pepper to taste.

8. If using a pizza stone, carefully transfer the pizza onto the preheated stone using a pizza peel.

9. Bake the pizza in the preheated oven for 12-15 minutes, or until the crust is golden brown and the cheese is bubbly.

10. Remove the pizza from the oven and let it cool for a few minutes before slicing.

11. Garnish with fresh basil leaves before serving.

Nutrition Information:

- Calories: 320

- Protein: 15g

- Carbohydrates: 35g

- Fat: 15g

- Fiber: 8g

- Sugar: 5g

- Portion Size: 1/6 of pizza

Chapter 5: Snacks and Appetizers

These easy-to-make treats are perfect for satisfying craving between meals or impressing guests at any gathering. From vibrant veggie sticks paired with creamy guacamole to crispy baked sweet potato fries, each recipe offers a burst o flavor and nutrition.

Guacamole with Veggie Sticks

Ingredients:

- 2 ripe avocados
- 1 lime, juiced
- 1/4 cup diced red onion
- 1 small tomato, diced
- 1/4 cup chopped fresh cilantro
- Salt and pepper to taste
- Assorted veggie sticks (carrots, celery, bell peppers

Instructions:

1. In a bowl, mash the avocados with lime juice unt smooth.

2. Stir in diced onion, tomato, and cilantro.

3. Season with salt and pepper to taste.

4. Serve with veggie sticks for dipping.

Nutrition Information:

- Calories: 120
- Protein: 2g
- Carbohydrates: 8g
- Fat: 10g
- Fiber: 6g
- Sugar: 1g
- Portion Size: 1/4 cup guacamole with veggie sticks

Hummus and Whole Grain Crackers

Ingredients:

- 1 can (15 oz) chickpeas, drained and rinsed
- 2 cloves garlic
- 3 tablespoons tahini
- 2 tablespoons lemon juice
- 2 tablespoons olive oil
- Salt and pepper to taste
- Whole grain crackers for serving

Instructions:

1. In a food processor, blend chickpeas, garlic, tahini, lemon juice, and olive oil until smooth.

2. Season with salt and pepper to taste.

3. Serve with whole grain crackers.

Nutrition Information:

- Calories: 140
- Protein: 5g
- Carbohydrates: 15g
- Fat: 7g
- Fiber: 4g
- Sugar: 1g
- Portion Size: 2 tablespoons hummus with crackers

Roasted Chickpeas

Ingredients:

- 1 can (15 oz) chickpeas, drained and rinsed
- 1 tablespoon olive oil
- 1 teaspoon paprika
- 1/2 teaspoon garlic powder
- Salt to taste

Instructions:

1. Preheat oven to 400°F (200°C).

2. Pat chickpeas dry with a paper towel and remove any loose skins.

3. In a bowl, toss chickpeas with olive oil, paprika, garlic powder, and salt.

4. Spread chickpeas in a single layer on a baking sheet.

5. Roast in the oven for 20-25 minutes, shaking the pan halfway through, until crispy.

6. Let cool before serving.

Nutrition Information:

- Calories: 120
- Protein: 5g
- Carbohydrates: 16g
- Fat: 4g
- Fiber: 5g
- Sugar: 1g
- Portion Size: 1/4 cup roasted chickpeas

Veggie Sushi Rolls

Ingredients:

- Nori sheets
- Cooked sushi rice
- Assorted vegetables (cucumber, avocado, carrot, bell pepper)
- Soy sauce and wasabi for dipping

Instructions:

1. Place a nori sheet on a bamboo sushi mat.
2. Spread a layer of cooked sushi rice evenly over the nori, leaving a border at the top.
3. Arrange thinly sliced vegetables along the bottom edge of the nori.
4. Roll the sushi tightly using the bamboo mat, sealing the edge with a little water.
5. Slice the roll into bite-sized pieces.
6. Serve with soy sauce and wasabi for dipping.

Nutrition Information:

- Calories: 110
- Protein: 2g

- Carbohydrates: 22g
- Fat: 1g
- Fiber: 3g
- Sugar: 1g
- Portion Size: 1 roll

Caprese Skewers

Ingredients:

- Cherry tomatoes
- Fresh mozzarella balls
- Fresh basil leaves
- Balsamic glaze for drizzling

Instructions:

1. Thread a cherry tomato, a mozzarella ball, and a basil leaf onto a small skewer.
2. Repeat with remaining ingredients.
3. Arrange skewers on a serving platter.
4. Drizzle with balsamic glaze before serving.

Nutrition Information:

- Calories: 60

- Protein: 3g
- Carbohydrates: 2g
- Fat: 4g
- Fiber: 1g
- Sugar: 1g
- Portion Size: 2 skewers

Edamame with Sea Salt

Ingredients:

- Frozen edamame in pods
- Coarse sea salt

Instructions:

1. Cook edamame according to package instructions.
2. Drain and pat dry with a paper towel.
3. Sprinkle with sea salt before serving.

Nutrition Information:

- Calories: 90
- Protein: 8g
- Carbohydrates: 8g
- Fat: 3g

- Fiber: 4g

- Sugar: 2g

- Portion Size: 1/2 cup edamame

aked Sweet Potato Fries

gredients:

- Sweet potatoes, cut into fries

- Olive oil

- Salt and pepper

structions:

1. Preheat oven to 425°F (220°C).

2. Toss sweet potato fries with olive oil, salt, and pepper.

3. Spread fries in a single layer on a baking sheet.

4. Bake for 25-30 minutes, flipping halfway through, until crispy.

5. Serve hot.

utrition Information:

- Calories: 120

- Protein: 2g

- Carbohydrates: 26g

- Fat: 2g

- Fiber: 4g

- Sugar: 5g

- Portion Size: 1 cup sweet potato fries

Cucumber and Cream Cheese Roll-Ups

Ingredients:

- English cucumber

- Cream cheese (regular or vegan)

- Smoked salmon (optional)

- Fresh dill or chives

Instructions:

1. Slice cucumber lengthwise into thin strips using vegetable peeler.

2. Spread a thin layer of cream cheese onto ea cucumber strip.

3. If using, place a small piece of smoked salmon on of the cream cheese.

4. Roll up the cucumber strip tightly.

5. Secure with a toothpick if necessary.

6. Garnish with fresh dill or chives before serving.

Nutrition Information:

- Calories: 40 (without smoked salmon)

- Protein: 1g

- Carbohydrates: 2g

- Fat: 3g

- Fiber: 1g

- Sugar: 1g

- Portion Size: 2 roll-ups

Stuffed Mushrooms with Herbs and Cheese

Ingredients:

- Large mushrooms, stems removed

- Cream cheese (regular or vegan)

- Fresh herbs (parsley, thyme, rosemary)

- Grated Parmesan cheese (optional)

- Olive oil

- Salt and pepper

Instructions:

1. Preheat oven to 375°F (190°C).
2. In a bowl, mix cream cheese with chopped fresh herbs and grated Parmesan cheese, if using.
3. Stuff each mushroom cap with the cream cheese mixture.
4. Drizzle with olive oil and season with salt and pepper.
5. Bake for 15-20 minutes until mushrooms are tender and cheese is golden.
6. Serve hot.

Nutrition Information:

- Calories: 60
- Protein: 3g
- Carbohydrates: 2g
- Fat: 5g
- Fiber: 1g
- Sugar: 1g
- Portion Size: 2 stuffed mushrooms

Greek Yogurt Dip with Veggies

Ingredients:

- Greek yogurt
- Garlic powder
- Dried dill
- Lemon juice
- Assorted raw vegetables (carrots, cucumber, bell peppers)

Instructions:

1. In a bowl, mix Greek yogurt with garlic powder, dried dill, and lemon juice to taste.
2. Stir until well combined.
3. Serve with assorted raw vegetables for dipping.

Nutrition Information:

- Calories: 70
- Protein: 5g
- Carbohydrates: 8g
- Fat: 2g
- Fiber: 2g
- Sugar: 5g

- Portion Size: 1/4 cup dip with veggies

Fruit and Cheese Platter

Ingredients:

- Assorted fruits (grapes, strawberries, apple slices)
- Assorted cheeses (cheddar, brie, goat cheese)
- Nuts (almonds, walnuts)
- Honey for drizzling (optional)

Instructions:

1. Arrange the fruits and cheeses on a serving platter.
2. Add nuts to the platter for extra crunch and flavor.
3. Drizzle honey over the cheeses if desired.
4. Serve as is or with whole grain crackers on the side

Nutrition Information:

- Calories: 150
- Protein: 7g
- Carbohydrates: 15g
- Fat: 8g
- Fiber: 3g
- Sugar: 10g

- Portion Size: 1/2 cup fruit and cheese

vocado Bruschetta

gredients:

- Baguette, sliced
- Ripe avocados
- Cherry tomatoes, diced
- Red onion, finely chopped
- Fresh basil, chopped
- Balsamic glaze
- Salt and pepper to taste

structions:

1. Toast the baguette slices until golden brown.
2. Mash the ripe avocados in a bowl and season with salt and pepper.
3. In another bowl, mix diced tomatoes, chopped red onion, and fresh basil.
4. Spread avocado mixture onto each baguette slice.
5. Top with tomato mixture and drizzle with balsamic glaze.
6. Serve immediately.

Nutrition Information:

- Calories: 120
- Protein: 3g
- Carbohydrates: 15g
- Fat: 6g
- Fiber: 3g
- Sugar: 2g
- Portion Size: 2 slices bruschetta

Spinach and Artichoke Dip with Whole Wheat Pita

Ingredients:

- Frozen spinach, thawed and drained
- Canned artichoke hearts, chopped
- Greek yogurt
- Cream cheese (regular or vegan)
- Garlic powder
- Shredded mozzarella cheese (optional)
- Whole wheat pita bread, cut into wedges

1. Preheat oven to 375°F (190°C).
2. In a bowl, mix together spinach, artichoke hearts, Greek yogurt, cream cheese, garlic powder, and shredded mozzarella cheese if using.
3. Transfer mixture to a baking dish and spread evenly.
4. Bake for 20-25 minutes until hot and bubbly.
5. Serve with whole wheat pita wedges for dipping.

Nutrition Information:

- Calories: 140
- Protein: 6g
- Carbohydrates: 18g
- Fat: 6g
- Fiber: 4g
- Sugar: 2g
- Portion Size: 1/4 cup dip with 2 pita wedges

Trail Mix with Nuts and Dried Fruit

Ingredients:

- Almonds
- Cashews

- Dried cranberries

- Dried apricots, chopped

- Dark chocolate chips (optional)

Instructions:

1. In a bowl, combine almonds, cashews, dried cranberries, dried apricots, and dark chocolate chips if using.

2. Mix well to distribute ingredients evenly.

3. Store in an airtight container for a quick and easy snack on the go.

Nutrition Information:

- Calories: 150

- Protein: 5g

- Carbohydrates: 15g

- Fat: 9g

- Fiber: 3g

- Sugar: 8g

- Portion Size: 1/4 cup trail mix

Greek Yogurt with Honey and Granola

Ingredients:

- Greek yogurt
- Honey
- Granola (store-bought or homemade)

Instructions:

1. Spoon Greek yogurt into a bowl.
2. Drizzle honey over the yogurt.
3. Sprinkle granola on top for added crunch and flavor.
4. Enjoy immediately as a satisfying snack or light dessert.

Nutrition Information:

- Calories: 200
- Protein: 15g
- Carbohydrates: 25g
- Fat: 6g
- Fiber: 2g
- Sugar: 15g
- Portion Size: 1 cup yogurt with toppings

Chapter 6: Desserts

These dessert recipes offer a perfect blend of flavors and textures, ensuring that you can enjoy a sweet treat without compromising your health. From fruity delights to creamy concoctions, each recipe is designed to tantalize your taste buds while keeping your blood sugar levels in check.

Berry Crisp with Oat Topping

Ingredients:

- 2 cups mixed berries (such as strawberries, blueberries, and raspberries)
- 1 tablespoon lemon juice
- 1/4 cup maple syrup
- 1/2 cup old-fashioned oats
- 1/4 cup almond flour
- 2 tablespoons coconut oil, melted
- 2 tablespoons chopped nuts (optional)

Instructions:

1. Preheat the oven to 350°F (175°C).

2. In a mixing bowl, toss the berries with lemon juice and maple syrup. Transfer the mixture to a baking dish.

3. In another bowl, combine oats, almond flour, coconut oil, and nuts (if using). Mix until crumbly.

4. Sprinkle the oat topping evenly over the berries.

5. Bake for 25-30 minutes, or until the topping is golden brown and the berries are bubbling.

6. Serve warm, optionally with a dollop of Greek yogurt or a scoop of vanilla ice cream.

utrition Information (per serving):

- Calories: 180
- Protein: 3g
- Carbohydrates: 25g
- Fat: 8g
- Fiber: 4g
- Sugar: 13g
- Portion Size: 1/6 of the crisp

Chocolate Avocado Mousse

Ingredients:

- 2 ripe avocados
- 1/4 cup cocoa powder
- 1/4 cup maple syrup or honey
- 1 teaspoon vanilla extract
- Pinch of salt
- Fresh berries, for garnish (optional)

Instructions:

1. In a food processor or blender, combine t
   avocados, cocoa powder, maple syrup, vani
   extract, and salt. Blend until smooth and creamy.
2. Transfer the mousse to serving glasses or bowls.
3. Chill in the refrigerator for at least 30 minutes befc
   serving.
4. Garnish with fresh berries, if desired, before servir

Nutrition Information (per serving):

- Calories: 180
- Protein: 2g
- Carbohydrates: 18g

- Fat: 12g

- Fiber: 6g

- Sugar: 9g

- Portion Size: 1/4 of the mousse

Banana Bread with Walnuts

Ingredients:

- 2 ripe bananas, mashed

- 1/4 cup coconut oil, melted

- 1/4 cup maple syrup or honey

- 1 teaspoon vanilla extract

- 2 cups whole wheat flour

- 1 teaspoon baking powder

- 1/2 teaspoon baking soda

- 1/2 teaspoon cinnamon

- 1/4 cup chopped walnuts

Instructions:

1. Preheat the oven to 350°F (175°C). Grease a loaf pan and set aside.

2. In a large mixing bowl, combine mashed bananas, coconut oil, maple syrup, and vanilla extract.

3. In a separate bowl, whisk together whole wheat flour, baking powder, baking soda, and cinnamon.

4. Gradually add the dry ingredients to the wet ingredients, stirring until just combined.

5. Fold in chopped walnuts.

6. Pour the batter into the prepared loaf pan and spread evenly.

7. Bake for 45-50 minutes, or until a toothpick inserted into the center comes out clean.

8. Allow the banana bread to cool in the pan for 10 minutes before transferring it to a wire rack to cool completely.

Nutrition Information (per serving):

- Calories: 180
- Protein: 4g
- Carbohydrates: 25g
- Fat: 8g
- Fiber: 4g
- Sugar: 10g
- Portion Size: 1 slice of banana bread

3. In another bowl, combine almond flour, rolled oats, chopped almonds, and melted coconut oil. Mix until crumbly.

4. Sprinkle the almond flour mixture evenly over the apples.

5. Bake for 30-35 minutes, or until the topping is golden brown and the apples are tender.

6. Allow the apple crisp to cool slightly before serving.

7. Serve warm, optionally with a scoop of vanilla ice cream or a dollop of Greek yogurt.

Nutrition Information (per serving):

- Calories: 200
- Protein: 4g
- Carbohydrates: 25g
- Fat: 10g
- Fiber: 5g
- Sugar: 16g
- Portion Size: 1/6 of the crisp

Greek Yogurt Berry Popsicles

Ingredients:

- 1 cup Greek yogurt
- 1 cup mixed berries (such as strawberries, blueberries, and raspberries)
- 2 tablespoons honey or maple syrup

Instructions:

1. In a blender, combine Greek yogurt, mixed berries, and honey or maple syrup. Blend until smooth.
2. Pour the mixture into popsicle molds, leaving a little space at the top for expansion.
3. Insert popsicle sticks into the molds.
4. Freeze for at least 4 hours, or until the popsicles are firm.
5. Run the molds under warm water for a few seconds to help release the popsicles.
6. Serve immediately or store in the freezer for later.

Nutrition Information (per serving):

- Calories: 80
- Protein: 5g

- Carbohydrates: 12g
- Fat: 2g
- Fiber: 2g
- Sugar: 9g
- Portion Size: 1 popsicle

Dark Chocolate Covered Strawberries

Ingredients:

- 1 cup dark chocolate chips
- 12 large strawberries, washed and dried

Instructions:

1. Line a baking sheet with parchment paper.
2. In a microwave-safe bowl, melt the dark chocolate chips in 30-second intervals, stirring in between, until smooth.
3. Holding each strawberry by the stem, dip it into the melted chocolate, coating it halfway.
4. Place the chocolate-covered strawberries on the prepared baking sheet.

5. Refrigerate for 20-30 minutes, or until the chocolate hardens.

6. Serve chilled.

Nutrition Information (per serving, 2 strawberries):

- Calories: 120
- Protein: 1g
- Carbohydrates: 16g
- Fat: 7g
- Fiber: 3g
- Sugar: 10g
- Portion Size: 2 strawberries

Baked Apples with Cinnamon and Nutmeg

Ingredients:

- 4 medium apples, cored
- 2 tablespoons maple syrup or honey
- 1 teaspoon cinnamon
- 1/2 teaspoon nutmeg

- 2 tablespoons chopped nuts (such as walnuts or pecans), optional

Instructions:

1. Preheat the oven to 375°F (190°C).
2. In a small bowl, mix together maple syrup or honey, cinnamon, and nutmeg.
3. Place the cored apples in a baking dish.
4. Fill each apple cavity with the maple syrup mixture.
5. Sprinkle chopped nuts over the top, if using.
6. Bake for 25-30 minutes, or until the apples are tender.
7. Serve warm, optionally with a scoop of Greek yogurt or a sprinkle of granola.

Nutrition Information (per serving, 1 apple):

- Calories: 140
- Protein: 1g
- Carbohydrates: 30g
- Fat: 3g
- Fiber: 5g
- Sugar: 23g
- Portion Size: 1 apple

Coconut Chia Seed Pudding

Ingredients:

- 1/4 cup chia seeds
- 1 cup coconut milk
- 1 tablespoon maple syrup or honey
- 1/2 teaspoon vanilla extract
- Fresh fruit, for topping (optional)

Instructions:

1. In a bowl, mix together chia seeds, coconut milk, maple syrup or honey, and vanilla extract.
2. Cover the bowl and refrigerate for at least 4 hours, or overnight, until the mixture thickens into pudding-like consistency.
3. Stir well before serving.
4. Top with fresh fruit, if desired, before serving.

Nutrition Information (per serving):

- Calories: 180
- Protein: 4g
- Carbohydrates: 15g
- Fat: 12g

- Fiber: 8g

- Sugar: 6g

- Portion Size: 1/2 cup of pudding

umpkin Pie Bites

gredients:

- 1 cup pumpkin puree

- 1/4 cup almond flour

- 2 tablespoons maple syrup or honey

- 1 teaspoon pumpkin pie spice

- 1/4 cup chopped pecans

- Whipped cream, for garnish (optional)

structions:

1. In a bowl, mix together pumpkin puree, almond flour, maple syrup or honey, and pumpkin pie spice until well combined.

2. Fold in chopped pecans.

3. Using a spoon, scoop out small portions of the mixture and roll into bite-sized balls.

4. Place the pumpkin pie bites on a baking sheet lined with parchment paper.

5. Chill in the refrigerator for at least 30 minutes befo
   serving.

6. Garnish with a dollop of whipped cream, if desire
   before serving.

Nutrition Information (per serving, 2 bites):

- Calories: 120
- Protein: 2g
- Carbohydrates: 10g
- Fat: 8g
- Fiber: 4g
- Sugar: 4g
- Portion Size: 2 bites

Almond Butter Cookies

Ingredients:

- 1 cup almond butter
- 1/4 cup maple syrup or honey
- 1 egg
- 1 teaspoon vanilla extract
- 1/2 teaspoon baking soda
- Pinch of salt

Instructions:

1. Preheat the oven to 350°F (175°C). Line a baking sheet with parchment paper.
2. In a mixing bowl, combine almond butter, maple syrup or honey, egg, vanilla extract, baking soda, and salt. Mix until well combined.
3. Scoop out tablespoon-sized portions of dough and roll into balls. Place them on the prepared baking sheet.
4. Use a fork to gently flatten each cookie and create a crisscross pattern on top.
5. Bake for 8-10 minutes, or until the edges are golden brown.
6. Allow the cookies to cool on the baking sheet for 5 minutes before transferring them to a wire rack to cool completely.

Nutrition Information (per serving, 2 cookies):

-   Calories: 160
-   Protein: 5g
-   Carbohydrates: 10g
-   Fat: 12g

- Fiber: 2g

- Sugar: 6g

- Portion Size: 2 cookies

Mango Sorbet

Ingredients:

- 2 cups frozen mango chunks

- 1/4 cup coconut water or water

- 1 tablespoon lime juice

- 1 tablespoon honey or maple syrup (optional)

Instructions:

1. In a blender, combine frozen mango chunks, coconut water or water, lime juice, and honey or maple syrup (if using).

2. Blend until smooth and creamy, scraping down the sides of the blender as needed.

3. Transfer the mixture to a shallow dish and spread it out evenly.

4. Freeze for at least 4 hours, or until firm.

5. Allow the sorbet to sit at room temperature for a few minutes before scooping and serving.

Nutrition Information (per serving):

- Calories: 90
- Protein: 1g
- Carbohydrates: 22g
- Fat: 0g
- Fiber: 2g
- Sugar: 20g
- Portion Size: 1/2 cup of sorbet

Carrot Cake Bites

Ingredients:

- 1 cup shredded carrots
- 1/2 cup rolled oats
- 1/4 cup chopped walnuts
- 1/4 cup raisins
- 2 tablespoons almond butter
- 1 tablespoon maple syrup or honey
- 1/2 teaspoon cinnamon
- Pinch of nutmeg

Instructions:

1. In a food processor, combine shredded carrots, rolled oats, chopped walnuts, raisins, almond butter, maple syrup or honey, cinnamon, and nutmeg.

2. Pulse until the mixture comes together and forms dough-like consistency.

3. Roll the mixture into bite-sized balls and place them on a plate or baking sheet.

4. Refrigerate for at least 30 minutes before serving.

Nutrition Information (per serving, 2 bites):

- Calories: 120
- Protein: 3g
- Carbohydrates: 15g
- Fat: 6g
- Fiber: 3g
- Sugar: 8g
- Portion Size: 2 bites

Frozen Yogurt Bark with Berries

Ingredients:

- 2 cups plain Greek yogurt

- 2 tablespoons honey or maple syrup
- 1 cup mixed berries (such as strawberries, blueberries, and raspberries)

Instructions:

1. In a bowl, mix together Greek yogurt and honey or maple syrup until well combined.
2. Line a baking sheet with parchment paper.
3. Spread the Greek yogurt mixture evenly onto the parchment paper, about 1/4 inch thick.
4. Sprinkle mixed berries evenly over the yogurt.
5. Freeze for at least 3 hours, or until firm.
6. Once frozen, break the yogurt bark into pieces.
7. Serve immediately or store in an airtight container in the freezer.

Nutrition Information (per serving):

- Calories: 70
- Protein: 6g
- Carbohydrates: 10g
- Fat: 0g
- Fiber: 1g

- Sugar: 8g

- Portion Size: 1/6 of the yogurt bark

Lemon Poppy Seed Muffins

Ingredients:

- 1 1/2 cups whole wheat flour

- 1/2 cup almond flour

- 1/2 cup maple syrup or honey

- 1/4 cup melted coconut oil

- 1/2 cup unsweetened applesauce

- 1/4 cup lemon juice

- Zest of 1 lemon

- 2 eggs

- 1 teaspoon baking powder

- 1/2 teaspoon baking soda

- 2 tablespoons poppy seeds

Instructions:

1. Preheat the oven to 350°F (175°C). Line a muffin
   with paper liners.

2. In a large bowl, whisk together whole wheat flour, almond flour, baking powder, baking soda, and poppy seeds.

3. In another bowl, mix together maple syrup or honey, melted coconut oil, applesauce, lemon juice, lemon zest, and eggs until well combined.

4. Gradually add the wet ingredients to the dry ingredients, stirring until just combined. Do not overmix.

5. Divide the batter evenly among the muffin cups, filling each about 3/4 full.

6. Bake for 18-20 minutes, or until a toothpick inserted into the center comes out clean.

7. Allow the muffins to cool in the tin for 5 minutes before transferring them to a wire rack to cool completely.

Nutrition Information (per serving, 1 muffin):

- Calories: 160
- Protein: 4g
- Carbohydrates: 20g
- Fat: 8g

- Fiber: 3g
- Sugar: 9g
- Portion Size: 1 muffin

These nutrient-packed blends are perfect for a quick and delicious breakfast, snack, or post-workout refuel. Packed with vitamins, minerals, and antioxidants, these smoothies are not only tasty but also provide a healthy boost to your day. Get ready to blend up some goodness!

Green Goddess Smoothie

Ingredients:

- 1 cup spinach
- 1/2 cup cucumber, chopped
- 1/2 avocado
- 1/2 banana
- 1/2 cup pineapple chunks
- 1 cup coconut water

Instructions:

1. Combine all ingredients in a blender.
2. Blend until smooth.
3. Serve immediately.

Nutrition Information:

- Calories: 180
- Protein: 4g
- Carbohydrates: 25g
- Fat: 9g
- Fiber: 7g
- Sugar: 15g
- Portion size: 1 serving

Blueberry Banana Smoothie

Ingredients:

- 1/2 cup blueberries
- 1 banana
- 1/2 cup Greek yogurt
- 1/2 cup almond milk
- Ice cubes (optional)

Instructions:

1. Combine all ingredients in a blender.
2. Blend until smooth.
3. Add ice cubes if desired and blend again.
4. Serve immediately.

Nutrition Information:

- Calories: 220
- Protein: 8g
- Carbohydrates: 35g
- Fat: 5g
- Fiber: 6g
- Sugar: 20g
- Portion size: 1 serving

Mango Coconut Smoothie

Ingredients:

- 1 cup mango chunks
- 1/2 banana
- 1/4 cup coconut milk
- 1/2 cup Greek yogurt
- 1/2 cup orange juice

Instructions:

1. Combine all ingredients in a blender.
2. Blend until smooth.
3. Serve immediately.

Nutrition Information:

- Calories: 240
- Protein: 6g
- Carbohydrates: 45g
- Fat: 6g
- Fiber: 4g
- Sugar: 30g
- Portion size: 1 serving

Spinach and Pineapple Smoothie

Ingredients:

- 1 cup spinach
- 1/2 cup pineapple chunks
- 1/2 banana
- 1/2 cup coconut water
- Ice cubes (optional)

Instructions:

1. Combine all ingredients in a blender.
2. Blend until smooth.
3. Add ice cubes if desired and blend again.
4. Serve immediately.

Nutrition Information:

- Calories: 160
- Protein: 3g
- Carbohydrates: 35g
- Fat: 1g
- Fiber: 5g
- Sugar: 20g
- Portion size: 1 serving

Berry Blast Smoothie

Ingredients:

- 1/2 cup strawberries
- 1/2 cup blueberries
- 1/2 cup raspberries
- 1/2 banana
- 1/2 cup almond milk
- Ice cubes (optional)

Instructions:

1. Combine all ingredients in a blender.
2. Blend until smooth.
3. Add ice cubes if desired and blend again.
4. Serve immediately.

Nutrition Information:

- Calories: 200
- Protein: 5g
- Carbohydrates: 40g
- Fat: 3g
- Fiber: 9g
- Sugar: 20g
- Portion size: 1 serving

Peanut Butter and Banana Smoothie

Ingredients:

- 1 banana
- 2 tablespoons peanut butter
- 1/2 cup Greek yogurt
- 1/2 cup almond milk
- Ice cubes (optional)

Instructions:

1. Combine all ingredients in a blender.
2. Blend until smooth.
3. Add ice cubes if desired and blend again.
4. Serve immediately.

Nutrition Information:

- Calories: 320
- Protein: 15g
- Carbohydrates: 30g
- Fat: 18g
- Fiber: 5g
- Sugar: 15g
- Portion size: 1 serving

Kale and Apple Smoothie

Ingredients:

- 1 cup kale leaves, stemmed and chopped
- 1 apple, cored and chopped
- 1/2 banana
- 1/2 cup almond milk
- 1 tablespoon honey (optional)
- Ice cubes (optional)

Instructions:

1. Combine all ingredients in a blender.
2. Blend until smooth.
3. Add honey if desired for sweetness.

4. Add ice cubes if desired and blend again.

5. Serve immediately.

Nutrition Information:

- Calories: 180

- Protein: 4g

- Carbohydrates: 35g

- Fat: 3g

- Fiber: 7g

- Sugar: 20g

- Portion size: 1 serving

Chocolate Peanut Butter Smoothie

Ingredients:

- 1 banana

- 2 tablespoons cocoa powder

- 2 tablespoons peanut butter

- 1/2 cup Greek yogurt

- 1/2 cup almond milk

- Ice cubes (optional)

structions:

1. Combine all ingredients in a blender.
2. Blend until smooth.
3. Add ice cubes if desired and blend again.
4. Serve immediately.

trition Information:

- Calories: 330
- Protein: 15g
- Carbohydrates: 30g
- Fat: 18g
- Fiber: 6g
- Sugar: 15g
- Portion size: 1 serving

aspberry Almond Smoothie

gredients:

- 1/2 cup raspberries
- 1/2 banana
- 1/4 cup almond butter
- 1/2 cup almond milk
- Ice cubes (optional)

Instructions:

1. Combine all ingredients in a blender.
2. Blend until smooth.
3. Add ice cubes if desired and blend again.
4. Serve immediately.

Nutrition Information:

- Calories: 280
- Protein: 8g
- Carbohydrates: 25g
- Fat: 18g
- Fiber: 7g
- Sugar: 10g
- Portion size: 1 serving

Orange Creamsicle Smoothie

Ingredients:

- 1 orange, peeled and segmented
- 1/2 banana
- 1/2 cup Greek yogurt
- 1/2 cup almond milk
- 1 tablespoon honey (optional)

- Ice cubes (optional)

Instructions:

1. Combine all ingredients in a blender.
2. Blend until smooth.
3. Add honey if desired for sweetness.
4. Add ice cubes if desired and blend again.
5. Serve immediately.

Nutrition Information:

- Calories: 200
- Protein: 7g
- Carbohydrates: 35g
- Fat: 3g
- Fiber: 5g
- Sugar: 25g
- Portion size: 1 serving

Avocado Spinach Smoothie

Ingredients:

- 1/2 avocado
- 1 cup spinach

- 1/2 banana

- 1/2 cup almond milk

- 1 tablespoon honey (optional)

- Ice cubes (optional)

Instructions:

1. Combine all ingredients in a blender.

2. Blend until smooth.

3. Add honey if desired for sweetness.

4. Add ice cubes if desired and blend again.

5. Serve immediately.

Nutrition Information:

- Calories: 220

- Protein: 5g

- Carbohydrates: 30g

- Fat: 11g

- Fiber: 7g

- Sugar: 15g

- Portion size: 1 serving

Peach and Ginger Smoothie

Ingredients:

- 1 peach, pitted and chopped
- 1/2 banana
- 1/2 inch piece of ginger, peeled and chopped
- 1/2 cup Greek yogurt
- 1/2 cup almond milk
- Ice cubes (optional)

Instructions:

1. Combine all ingredients in a blender.
2. Blend until smooth.
3. Add ice cubes if desired and blend again.
4. Serve immediately.

Nutrition Information:

- Calories: 210
- Protein: 7g
- Carbohydrates: 40g
- Fat: 4g
- Fiber: 6g
- Sugar: 25g

- Portion size: 1 serving

Turmeric Mango Smoothie

Ingredients:

- 1 cup mango chunks
- 1/2 banana
- 1/2 teaspoon turmeric powder
- 1/2 teaspoon ginger powder
- 1/2 cup coconut milk
- Ice cubes (optional)

Instructions:

1. Combine all ingredients in a blender.
2. Blend until smooth.
3. Add ice cubes if desired and blend again.
4. Serve immediately.

Nutrition Information:

- Calories: 250
- Protein: 4g
- Carbohydrates: 40g
- Fat: 9g

- Fiber: 5g
- Sugar: 25g
- Portion size: 1 serving

ucumber Mint Smoothie

gredients:

- 1/2 cucumber, peeled and chopped
- 1/4 cup fresh mint leaves
- 1/2 cup Greek yogurt
- 1/2 cup coconut water
- 1 tablespoon honey (optional)
- Ice cubes (optional)

tructions:

1. Combine all ingredients in a blender.
2. Blend until smooth.
3. Add honey if desired for sweetness.
4. Add ice cubes if desired and blend again.
5. Serve immediately.

trition Information:

- Calories: 150

- Protein: 6g

- Carbohydrates: 25g

- Fat: 2g

- Fiber: 3g

- Sugar: 20g

- Portion size: 1 serving

Beet Berry Smoothie

Ingredients:

- 1/2 cup cooked beets, chopped

- 1/2 cup mixed berries (strawberries, blueberries, raspberries)

- 1/2 banana

- 1/2 cup almond milk

- Ice cubes (optional)

Instructions:

1. Combine all ingredients in a blender.

2. Blend until smooth.

3. Add ice cubes if desired and blend again.

4. Serve immediately.

Nutrition Information:

- Calories: 200
- Protein: 5g
- Carbohydrates: 40g
- Fat: 2g
- Fiber: 9g
- Sugar: 25g
- Portion size: 1 serving

CONCLUSION

"Gestational Diabetes Recipes for Vegetarians" offers a holistic approach to managing gestational diabetes through delicious and nutritious vegetarian meals. Throughout this book, we've explored a diverse array of recipes carefully crafted to meet the dietary needs of expecting mothers while ensuring optimal blood sugar control.

By embracing the principles of vegetarianism and incorporating wholesome ingredients rich in fiber, vitamins and minerals, this collection provides not only sustenance but also culinary delight. From hearty breakfasts to satisfying dinners, from wholesome snacks to indulgent desserts, each recipe is thoughtfully designed to support maternal health and well-being during this transformative phase of life.

Beyond the kitchen, this book serves as a guide, empowering mothers-to-be with knowledge and tools to navigate gestational diabetes with confidence. By following the 30 day meal plan or selecting recipes to suit individual taste and preferences, readers can embark on a journey of culinary exploration while prioritizing their health and the health of their baby.

As we conclude this culinary journey, let us remember that managing gestational diabetes is not merely about restriction, but rather about embracing a lifestyle of balance and nourishment. By nourishing our bodies with wholesome, plant-based foods and embracing mindful eating habits, we can foster a sense of well-being that extends far beyond pregnancy.

May this book serve as a companion on your path to wellness, offering inspiration, support, and encouragement as you nourish yourself and your growing baby with love, compassion, and the vibrant flavors of vegetarian cuisine. Here's to a journey filled with health, happiness, and delicious meals shared with loved ones. Cheers to you and your beautiful journey through motherhood!